Delicious Recipes for Bariatric Diet

Bariatric Diet

Lunch

Healthy food sources

Megan Spark

Table of Contents

Introduction

Gastric sleeve surgery is one of the most effective ways of losing weight. It is a type of bariatric surgery that involves altering your stomach and small intestine to absorb and digest small amounts of food. It leads to 60-80 percent excess weight loss and provides an excellent resolution of many obesity-relation health issues such as high blood pressure, type 2 diabetes, sleep apnea and joint pain.

But after this quick and life-saving procedure is the need to the stop the behaviors that led to the obesity in the first place. It is essential to create new habits, and maintain long term changes. In fact, you need a complete change of lifestyle to enjoy long-lasting success.

This isn't as easy as it seem, because it's hard to change a bad habit and build the right one. Changing your diet is the first step. It is essential that you know what you eat and what you can't eat as the weeks progresses. The first 5 weeks is extremely important because eating the wrong foods can worsen your healing stomach. But eating the right foods and in the right amounts will enable your body heal faster.

In the first few weeks, you can only take liquids and small amounts of small foods. Most times only 2 tablespoons of food is all it takes to feel full. Eating solid food is a gradual process that is started within 2 months. Even then, you will feel full very quickly. You may require nutritional supplements as well.

You will continue to lose weight for about a year before stabilizing. You will lose 1/2 or 2/3rd of excess body weight eventually. Consistent monitoring of your food intake by tracking and measuring what you eat also help to sustain weight loss. Have a food journal or use an online diary to do this. You may also count calories. Furthermore, keep in touch with your dietitian or nutritionist.

And you must exercise! Exercise is a vital component of weight loss. Having an exercise plan and sticking with it will activate more excess weight loss. Have a scheduled time for exercise. Join group classes to make it easier for you. Use personal trainers if you can afford it. How fast you lose weight depends on you. Besides, being fit will make you look good and feel good. So establish fitness goals. It is more beneficial than having only scale-based weight loss goals.

1. **<u>Cold Tomato Couscous</u>**

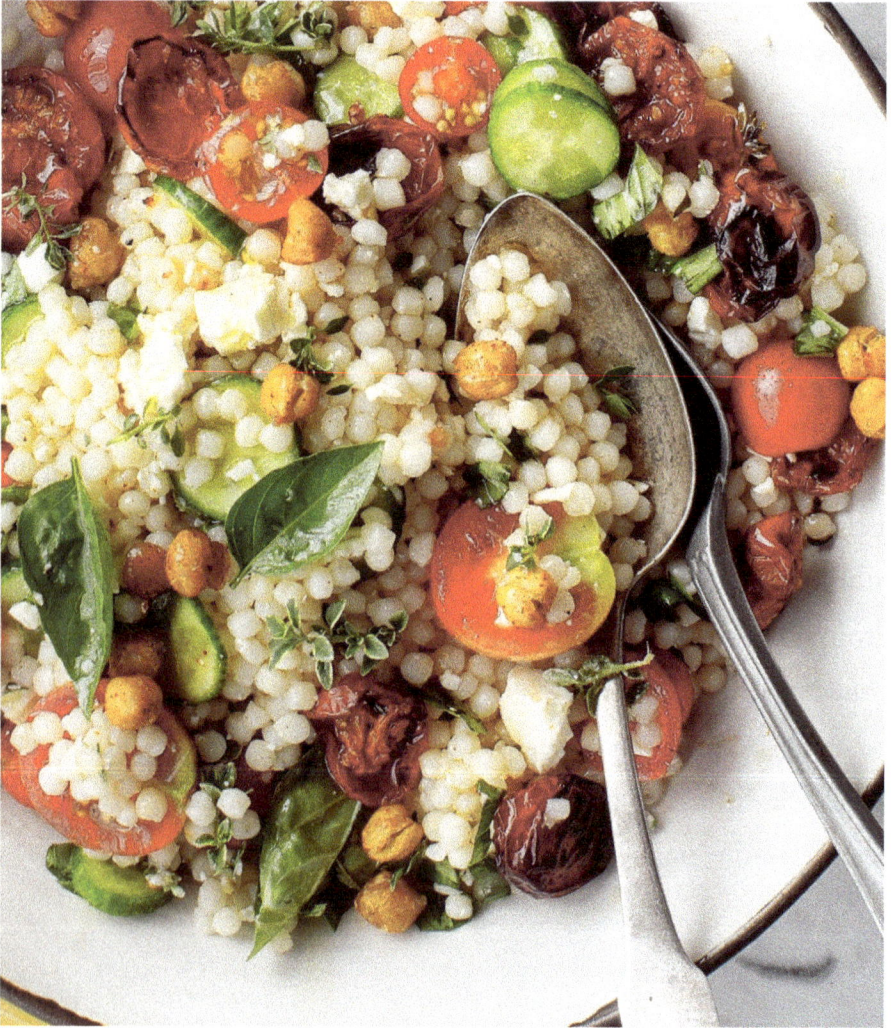

Serves: 4

Preparation time: 15 minutes

Cooking time: 7-10 minutes

Ingredients:

- 5 oz couscous
- 3 tbsp tomato sauce
- 3 tbsp lemon juice
- 1 small-sized onion, chopped
- 1 cup vegetable stock
- ½ small-sized cucumber, sliced
- ½ small-sized carrot, sliced
- ¼ tsp salt
- 3 tbsp olive oil
- ½ cup fresh parsley, chopped

Preparation:

1. First, pour the couscous into a large bowl. Boil the vegetable broth and slightly add in the couscous while stirring constantly.
2. Leave it for about 10 minutes until couscous absorbs the iquid. Cover with a lid and set aside. Stir from time to time to speed up the soaking process and break the lumps with a spoon.
3. Meanwhile, preheat the olive oil in a frying pan, and add the tomato sauce.
4. Add chopped onion and stir until translucent. Set aside and let it cool for a few minutes.
5. Add the oily tomato sauce to the couscous and stir well.

6. Now add lemon juice, chopped parsley, and salt to the mixture and give it a final stir.

7. Serve with sliced cucumber, carrot, and parsley.

Nutrition information per serving: Calories: 249, Protein: 5.6g, Total Carbs: 32.8g, Dietary Fibers: 3.2g, Total Fat: 11g

2. **Wild Salmon Salad**

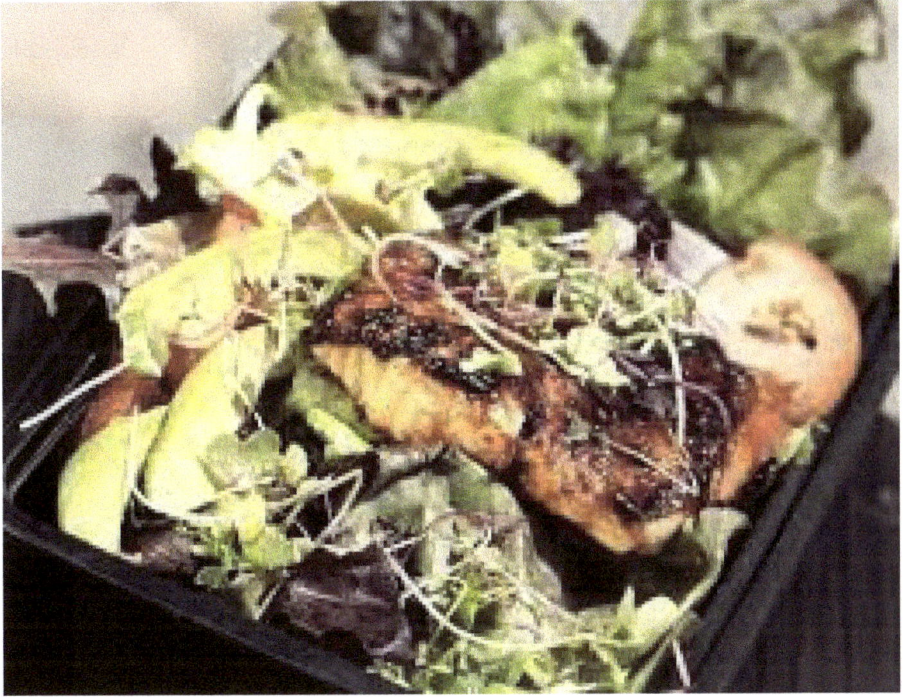

Serves: 2

Preparation time: 10 minutes

Cooking time: -

Ingredients:

- 2 medium-sized cucumbers, sliced
- A handful of iceberg lettuce, torn
- ¼ cup sweet corn
- 1 large tomato, roughly chopped

- 8 oz smoked wild salmon, sliced
- 4 tbsp freshly squeezed orange juice

Dressing:

- 1 ¼ cup liquid yogurt, 2% fat
- 1 tbsp fresh mint, finely chopped
- 2 garlic cloves, crushed
- 1 tbsp sesame seeds

Preparation:

1. Combine vegetables in a large bowl.
2. Drizzle with orange juice and top with salmon slices.
3. Set aside. In another bowl, whisk together yogurt, mint, crushed garlic, and sesame seeds.
4. Drizzle over salad and toss to combine.
5. Serve cold.

Nutrition information per serving: Calories: 249, Protein: 5.6g, Total Carbs: 32.8g, Dietary Fibers: 3.2g, Total Fat: 11g

3. Quinoa Bowls

Prep Time: 10 minutes

Cook Time: 25 minutes

Servings: 2

Ingredients

Vegetables:

- 8 oz. asparagus stalks
- 11/2 cups cauliflower florets
- 11/2 cups radishes, halved
- 1 tablespoon olive oil
- 1/2 tablespoon seasoning

Sauce:

- ½ tablespoon tahini
- 2 tablespoons lemon juice
- ¼ teaspoon garlic powder
- ½ teaspoon turmeric
- ¼ teaspoon of pepper flakes
- Salt & pepper

Bowls:

- Roasted veggies
- 11/2 cups of cooked quinoa
- 1 cup arugula
- 1 avocado

Preparation:

1. Preheat oven to 400F. Spritz baking sheet with cooking spray.

2. Trim off asparagus ends. Add to the baking sheet, as well as the cauliflower and radishes. Drizzle with oil, sprinkle with seasoning of choice and stir.

3. Place in the oven and cook, flipping halfway, until lightly browned. This should take about 25 minutes. Flip halfway through to ensure even cooking.

4. Whisk dressing ingredients together. Thin the sauce with water. Do this gradually until the texture is drizzly.

5. Assemble the bowls and divide ingredients evenly. Refrigerate along with the serve.

6. When ready to eat, top with the sauce and the sliced avocado.

Nutrition Per Serving: Calories: 396kcal | Fat: 19g | Carbs: 47g | Protein: 12g| Fiber 13g| Sodium 80mg| Cholesterol 8mg

4. <u>Black Bean Salsa</u>

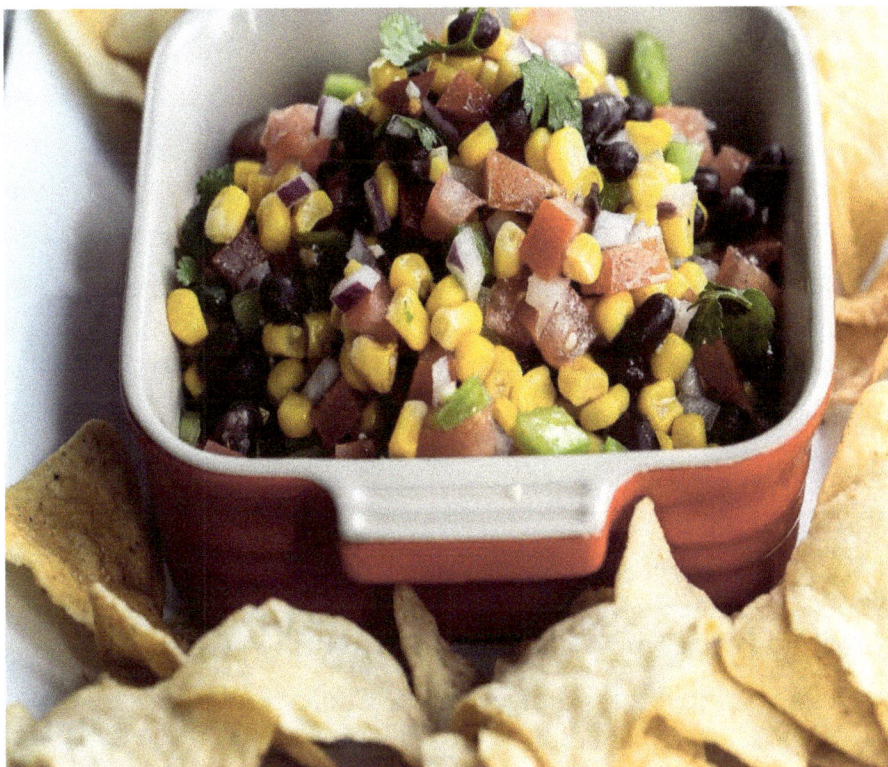

Prep/Total Time: 20 minutes

Servings:3-1/2 cups

- Diet Phase: Soft food
- Ingredients:
- 1 15- ounce can black beans, rinsed and drained
- 1 medium cucumber, seeded chopped
- ½ cup of chopped tomato
- ½ cup of green onions, sliced

- ¼ cup of lime juice
- 1 tablespoon of snipped fresh cilantro
- 1 tablespoon of olive oil
- ½ teaspoon ground cumin
- 1/3 teaspoon salt
- 1/3 teaspoon cayenne pepper

Preparation:

1. Add together all the ingredients in a bowl, cover and refrigerate for 4 hours.

2. Enjoy over grilled meat.

3. Make ahead: refrigerate, covered, for up to 24 hours.

Nutrition Per Serving Calories: 35kcal | Fat: 1g | Carbs: 6g | Protein: 2g| Fiber 2g| 98 mg sodium| Cholesterol 0mg

5. <u>Caesar Salad</u>

Prep Time: 10 minutes

Cook Time: 10 minutes

Servings: 3

Ingredients:

- Croutons:
- ½ tablespoon olive oil
- ¾ - 1 cup bread cubes (a day-old)
- 1/4 teaspoon of kosher salt

Dressing:

- ¼ (2 oz.) can anchovy fillets, oil-packed, drained
- 1 small cloves garlic, chopped coarsely
- 1 large egg yolk
- 1/4 teaspoon Dijon mustard
- 1/2 tablespoon fresh lemon juice
- ½ tablespoon olive oil
- 2 tablespoons of vegetable oil
- 1 tablespoon Parmesan cheese, finely grated
- Freshly ground black pepper

Salad:

- 3/4 medium hearts romaine lettuce
- 1 oz. Parmesan cheese, shaved with a vegetable peeler

Preparation:

1. Add oil to pan and heat and once hot, add the bread cubes, sprinkle with salt and stir to coat with the oil. Toast and toss the bread cubes for 5 minutes until golden brown. Remove and let it cool.

2. Mix the garlic and anchovies together until paste-like.

3. Whisk the egg yolk in a bowl. Add the mustard and whisk. Add the anchovygarlic mixture. Whisk. Add the lemon juice and whisk to mix all.

4. Now add the olive oil and whisk to thicken for a minute or less. Pour in the vegetable oil and add the cheese. Season with black pepper.

5. Cut the romaine into pieces, rinse and pat dry.

6. Place the romaine in a bowl, add ½ of the dressing and mix.Add the croutons, toss and add some more cheese and pepper as needed.

7. Make ahead:

Make croutons 3 days ahead and store at room temperature in an airtight container for up to 1 week.

Store in the freezer for up to 6 months. Store the leftover dressing in the refrigerator for up to a week.

Nutrition Per Serving Calories: 591kcal | Fat: 43g | Carbs: 15g | Protein: 30g| Fiber 2g| 2130mg sodium| Cholesterol 148mg

6. Baked Chicken Pesto

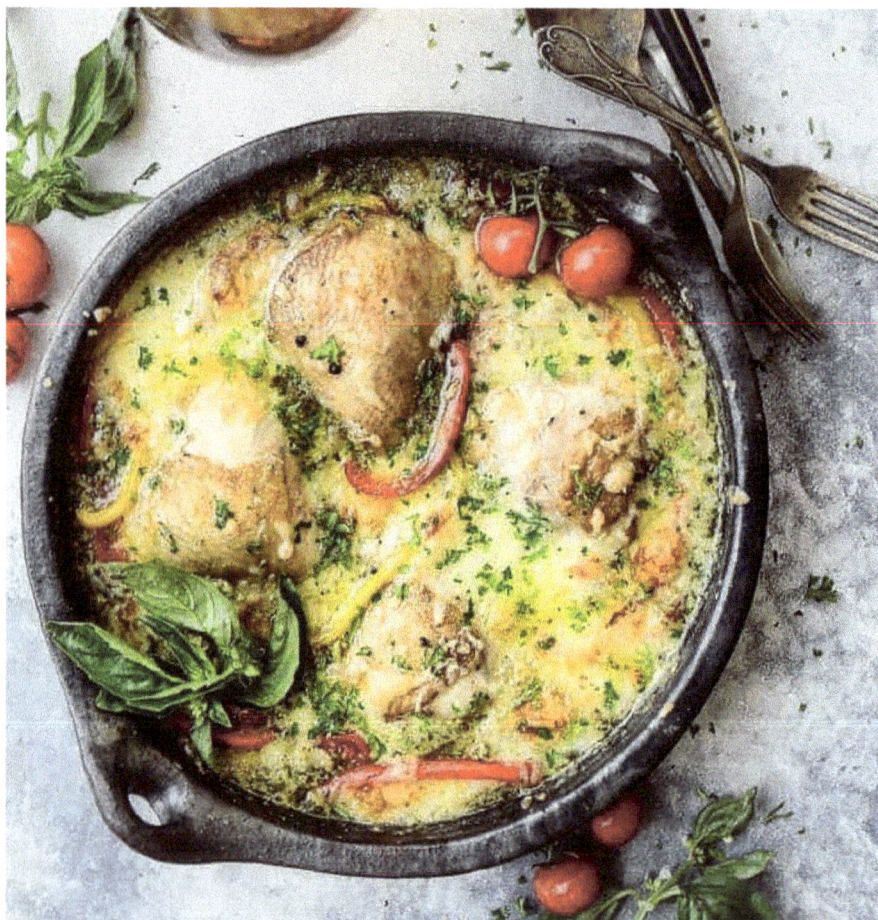

Prep Time: 10 minutes

Cook Time: 30 minutes

Servings: 2

Ingredients:

- 2 teaspoons of basil pesto
- 1 small tomatoes, thinly sliced
- 1 lb. chicken breasts, boneless & skinless
- 3 tablespoons of mozzarella cheese, shredded
- 1 teaspoon of parmesan cheese, grated
- Kosher salt and fresh pepper to taste

Preparation:

1. Preheat your oven to 400F; next line a large baking sheet with foil.

2. Make 2 very thin cutlets of chicken by slicing it horizontally, place the chicken in a large bowl and sprinkle with salt and pepper to season.

3. Place chicken on the foil-lined baking sheet, arrange well and spoon a teaspoon of pesto over each chicken piece. Bake for 25 minutes in the oven.

4. Remove, top with tomatoes and cheeses. Return to the oven to melt cheese.

Nutrition Per Serving Calories: 205kcal | Fat: 11g | Carbs: 2.5g | Protein: 30g| Fiber 0.5g|Sodium: 171.5mg | Cholesterol 90.5mg

7. **Slow Cooker Chicken**

Prep time: 10 minutes

Cook time: 4 hours

Servings: 6

INGREDIENTS

- 3 cup of cauliflower rice
- 1 tbsp of water
- 1 tbsp of corn starch
- 1 cup of low-sodium chicken broth
- 2 cup of light coconut milk
- 1 tsp of garlic minced
- 3 tbsp of curry powder
- 1 cup of frozen peas
- 1 large carrot diced
- 1 red bell pepper, cut into strips
- 1 medium yellow onion, cut into slices
- 1/4 tsp of each salt and pepper
- 1 pounds of skinless, boneless chicken thighs

INSTRUCTIONS

1. Sprinkle the chicken with salt and pepper.

2. Place chicken, carrots, bell pepper, peas, curry powder, garlic and onion in a slow cooker. Add the coconut milk and chicken broth and cook for 4 hours on low.

3. Remove chicken with a spoon from cooker onto a plate and gently shred.

4. Add water to a small mixing bowl, add the cornstarch and blend well until a paste forms.

5. Pour the cornstarch mix into the slow cooker and stir. Cook for about 10 minutes, and then place back the chicken. Cook further for an hour. Serve hot across cauliflower rice.

Nutrition per servings:

Calories: 330kcal; Carbohydrates: 9g; Protein: 23g; Fat: 19g

8. Tilapia Parmesan Crusted Zucchini

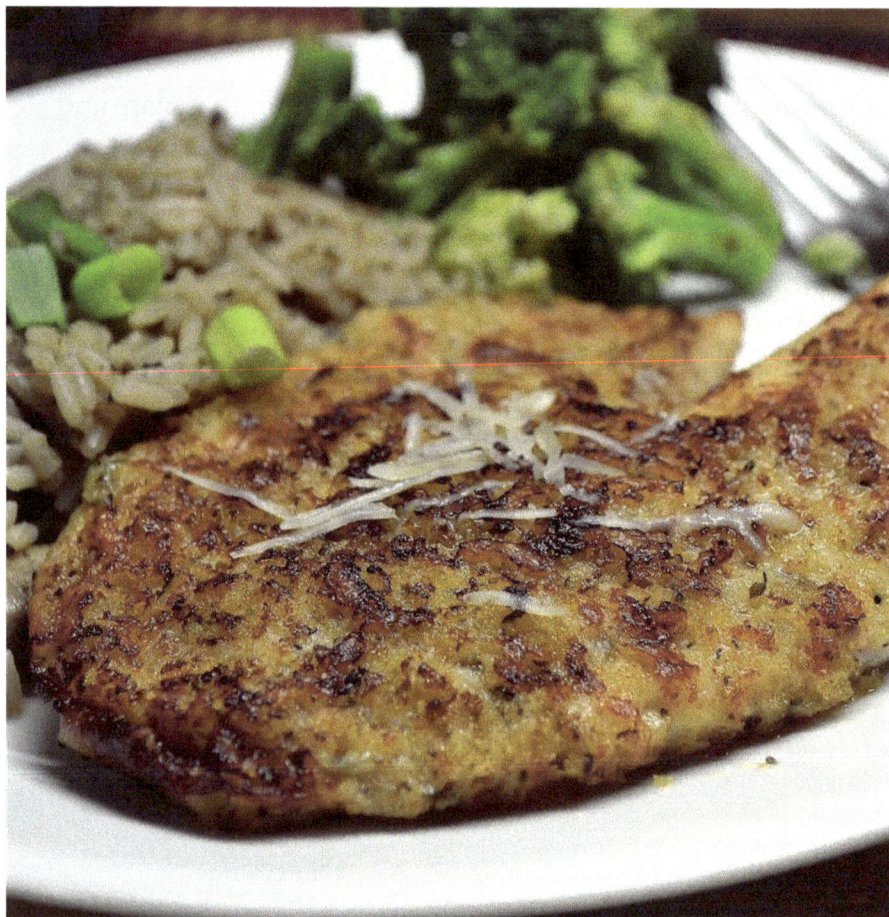

Prep time: 10 minutes

Cook time: 15 minutes

Servings: 2

INGREDIENTS

For the Tilapia

- 1 tbsp of capers
- 1 tsp of garlic minced
- 1 large lemon juiced
- 1/4 cup of Champagne vinegar (or white cooking wine)
- 1/2 tbsp of butter
- 1 tbsp of all-purpose flour (or cornstarch)
- Salt and pepper to taste
- 2 tilapia filets thawed if frozen
- 1 tbsp of extra-virgin olive oil

For the Parmesan crusted zucchini

- Non-stick cooking spray
- 2 eggs
- 1/2 cup of grated Parmesan cheese
- 1 medium zucchini cut 1/4 inch thick rounds

INSTRUCTIONS

Make the Tiliapia

1. Heat a frying pan over medium heat, generously spray with non-stick spray.

2. Season the tilapia filets all over with pepper and salt. Place in the pan and cook on each side for about 2 minutes. Remove and set aside.

3. Reduce to low heat, add the butter and flour and whisk until it simmering and starting to thicken. Add the lemon juice, Champagne vinegar and garlic, whisking for about 2-3 minutes.

4. Add in the capers and cook for additional 1-2 minutes. Taste and adjust with either 1 teaspoon of milk or butter. This will help calm it down if it makes you pucker. Spread sauce over fish to serve.

Make the zucchini

5. Place the eggs and cheese in different bowls.

6. Dredge each round of zucchini in the bowl of cheese, then dip in the egg bowl, then dip inside the cheese again.

7. Heat a frying pan over medium heat, generously spray with non-stick spray.

8.Cook the zuchinni in hot pan about 2-3 minutes on both sides.

9.Let it cook for more than half of the total time before flipping to allow the crust stick.

Transfer the zucchini and let drain on a paper towel before serving

9. <u>Zucchini Ravioli</u>

Prep time: 15 minutes

Cook time: 30 minutes

Servings: 4

INGREDIENTS

- Optional: Additional Italian-blend shredded cheese
- 2 medium zucchini, slice in 1/8 inch thick strips, length-wise
- 1 tsp of Italian seasoning
- ½ cup of grated parmesan cheese
- 2 cup of part-skim ricotta cheese
- 1 tbsp of tomato paste
- ½ tsp of cinnamon ½ tsp. nutmeg
- 15 ounces can of pumpkin puree (different from pumpkin pie filling)
- Salt and pepper, to taste
- 1 pounds of lean ground turkey
- 1 minced garlic clove
- I small sliced onion

INSTRUCTIONS

1. Heat-up the oven to 350 F.

2. Heat a frying pan over medium heat, generously spray with non-stick spray.

Sauté the onions in the hot skillet for 1-2 minutes it's soft. Add the ground turkey, garlic, salt, Italian seasoning and pepper and cook until ground turkey is browned.

3. Add the canned pumpkin, nutmeg and cinnamon, and stir well then add in tomato paste. Mix once again, reduce to low heat, cover and let simmer on low.

4. Combine the Parmesan cheese, ricotta cheese, pepper, Italian seasoning and salt in a bowl. Mix until well mixed.

5. Assemble the ravioli by laying out 2 slices of zucchini to form a plus sign. Add the ricotta/Parmesan mixture generously over the middle of the zucchini slices; fold the zucchini, starting from bottom, then the top. Place in an 8 x 8 casserole dish lying upside down. Repeat with the remaining. Top with pumpkin mixture.

9. Bake at 350 degrees F for 30 minutes in the oven. Top with more cheese, if needed.

Nutrition per servings:

Calories: 342kcal; Carbohydrates: 17g; Protein: 29g; Fat: 15g

10. <u>Broccoli Tofu Mushrooms Quiche</u>

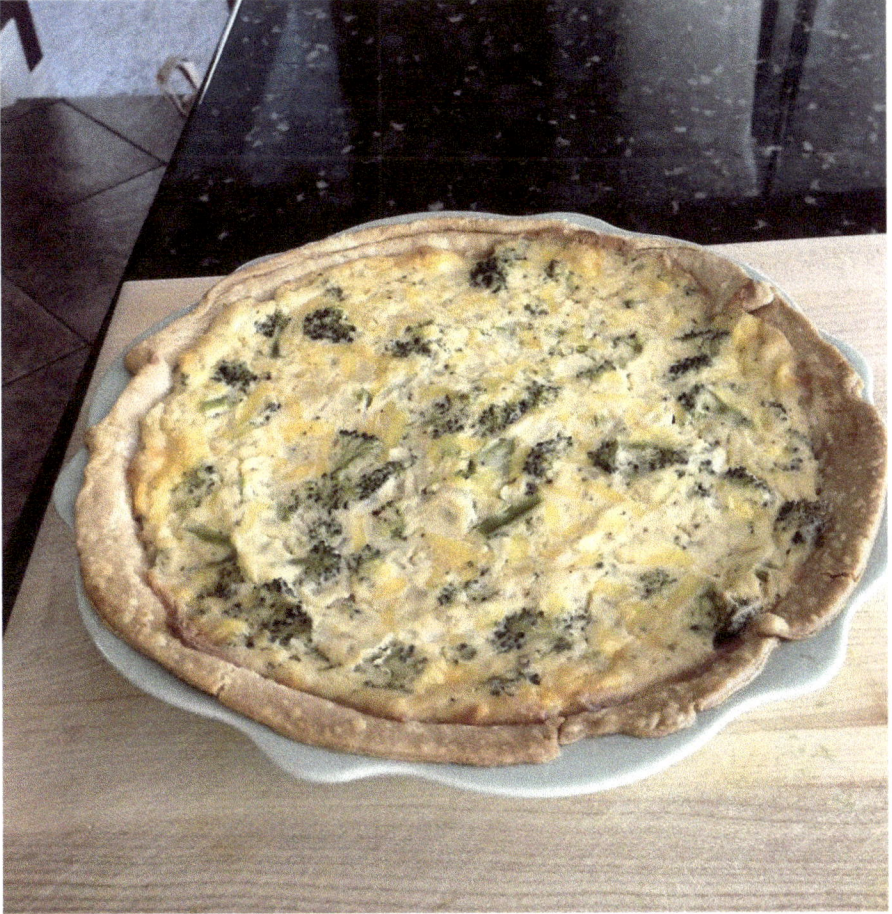

Prep time: 20 minutes

Cook time: 60 minutes

Servings: 6

INGREDIENTS

- 1 tbsp of tamari

- 1 tbsp of pickled plum paste or white miso
- 2 tbsp of sesame tahini
- 1½ lbs of tofu
- ¼ lb of chopped mushrooms
- ½ lb of chopped broccoli
- 1 yellow onion, chopped
- 1 tbsp of sesame oil
- Pinch of salt
- ½ cup of uncooked bulgur wheat

INSTRUCTIONS

1. Heat-up the oven to 350 F. Greased a 9-inch pie pan with non stick spray.

2. Add bulgur and a pinch of salt to 1 cup of boiling water in a small pot, return to a boil. Reduce heat and cook covered for 15 minutes.

3. Add the hot bulgur to the prepared pan, slightly press down and baked at 350 F for 12 minutes, or until kind of dry and a bit crusty. Set aside.

4. Heat the oil over medium high heat in a large skillet. Add onions, mushrooms and broccoli to the pan and cook briefly. Cover with a lid and remove from heat; set aside.

Prepare The Tofu Mixture

5. In a food processor, blend together the tofu, umeboshi paste, tamari and sesame tahini until smooth.

6. Combine the cooked vegetables and tofu mixture in a bowl. Gently toss to combine.

7. Add the vegetable tofu mixture onto the bulgur crust. Place pie pan in the oven and bake for 30 minutes. Remove and set aside for 10 minutes. Slice into 6 and serve.

Nutrition per servings:

Calories: 190kcal; Carbohydrates: 14g; Protein: 13g; Fat: 8g

11. Turkey Kickoff

Prep time: 15 minutes

Cook time: 15 minutes

Servings: 24 (2 per servings)

INGREDIENTS

- 3 (8 in each tube) tubes of refrigerated crescent rolls, reduced fat
- 1 cup of shredded 2% low fat cheese
- 1 lb of ground turkey (breast meat only)
- 1 envelope of dry onion soup

INSTRUCTIONS

1. Heat-up the oven to 350 F.

2. Mix the ground turkey meat and dry onion soup together in skillet and brown. Add in the cheese and mix well until finely blended.

3. Unroll and separate each crescent rolls, cut each triangle into half.

4. Spoon 1 tablespoon of meat mixture in middle of each of the triangle. Fold and seal the edges.

5. Place triangle on a cookie sheet and bake for 15 minutes

Nutrition per servings:

Calories: 155kcal; Carbohydrates: 13g; Protein: 9g; Fat: 7g

12. Chicken Philly Cheese Steak Sandwich

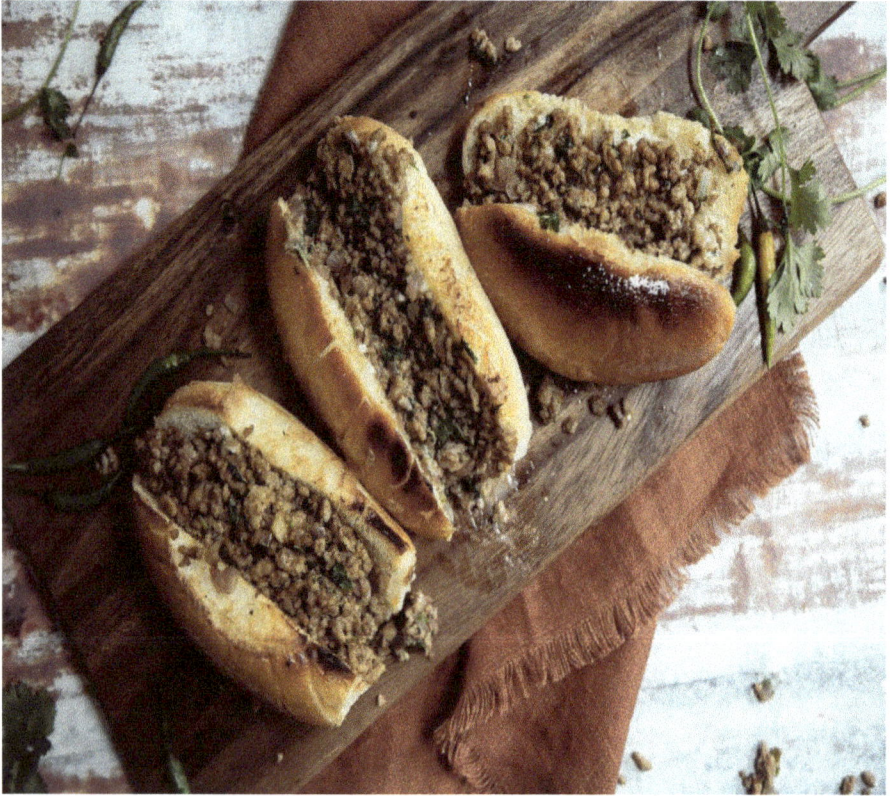

Prep Time: 10 minutes

Cook Time: 15 minutes

Serves: 2

Ingredients:

- 2 teaspoon of oil

- ¾ lb of boneless & skinless chicken breast, sliced thinly
- 1 clove of minced garlic
- ½ teaspoon of ground paprika
- 6 oz mushrooms, sliced thinly
- 1 tablespoon of unsalted butter
- ½ green pepper, sliced thinly
- ½ large onion, sliced thinly
- ½ teaspoon of ground black pepper
- 4 oz of sliced provolone cheese
- 1 teaspoon of salt
- 2 hoagie sandwich rolls
- Mayo, optional

Instructions:

1. Heat oil in a skillet over medium heat. Add chicken, sauté until cooked and browned. Remove from heat and set aside.

2. Melt the butter in the same skillet; add mushroom, onions, pepper and sauté for a few minutes until desired doneness.

3. Next stir in minced garlic, seasonings and chicken, cook until the garlic is fragrant.

4. Add cheese and cook covered for a few minutes until the cheese melts, remove from heat and set aside.

5. Toast the buns, spread with mayo and fill with cheese steak mixture, enjoy!

Nutrition per Serving

Calories: 669kcalCarbohydrates: 41gProtein: 71gFat: 24gSaturated Fat: 11g Cholesterol: 184mg

13. <u>Cabbage Rolls Without Rice</u>

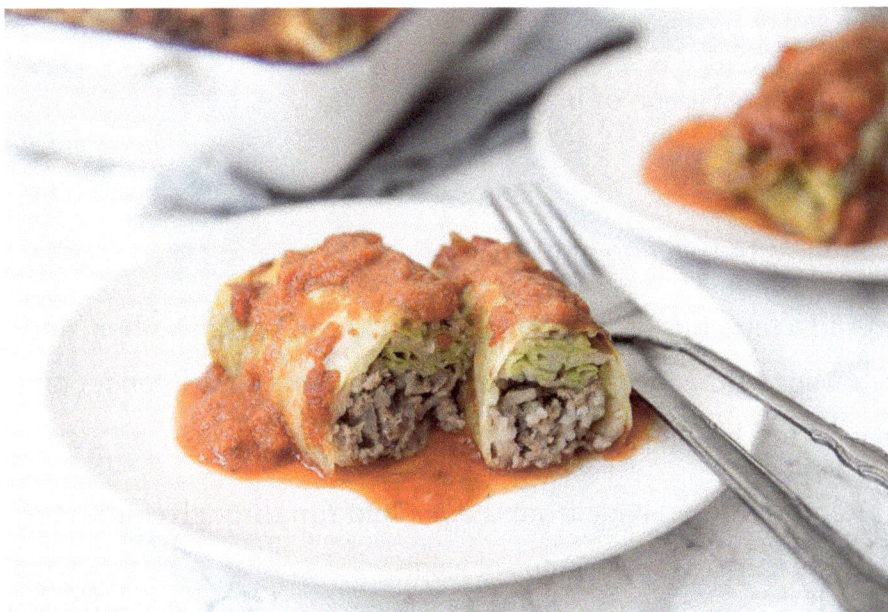

Prep Time: 30 minutes

Cook Time: 60 minutes

Serves: 6

Ingredients:

- 1 head of Cabbage
- 1 large egg, beaten
- 1 cup of cauliflower rice
- 1 15-oz can of tomato sauce
- 1 pound of ground beef

- 1 teaspoon of sea salt
- 4 cloves of minced garlic
- 2 teaspoon of Italian seasoning
- 1 14.5-oz can Diced tomatoes (drained)
- 1/4 teaspoon of Black pepper

Instructions:

1. Preheat the oven to 350F.

2. Add a few cups of water in a saucepan and bring to a boil, add cabbage to the saucepan and cook for 5 minutes until tender and leaves turn bright green.

3. Remove the cabbage from the pot and run through cold water, peel the cabbage leaves and set aside.

4. Cook cauliflower rice per package instructions, set aside.

5. Next, combine the ground beef, garlic, Italian seasoning, diced tomatoes, egg, salt and pepper in a large mixing bowl. Add cauliflower rice to the bowl and set aside.

6. Divide the tomato sauce in two, spread half of the tomato sauce in a large baking dish and set aside.

7. Cut a "V" shape in the center of each cabbage leaf, divide beef mixture into a log shape at the end of a cabbage leaf, fold and roll like a burrito. Repeat with the remaining cabbage rolls.

8. Place cabbage rolls seam side down in the baking dish, spoon the remaining tomato sauce over the cabbage rolls. Tent the baking dish tightly with foil, place in the oven and bake for 1 hour until cooked through.

Nutrition per Serving

Calories321, Fat18g, Protein25g, Total Carbs15g, Fiber5g, Sugar7g

14. **Baked Chicken Pesto**

Prep Time: 10 minutes

Cook Time: 30 minutes

Serves: 4

Ingredients:

- 4 teaspoons of basil pesto
- 1 medium tomatoes, sliced thin
- 2 16 oz chicken breasts, boneless & skinless
- 6 tablespoons of shredded mozzarella cheese
- 2 teaspoons of parmesan cheese, grated
- Kosher salt and fresh pepper to taste

Instructions:

1. Preheat the oven to 400F, line a large baking sheet with foil and set aside.

2. Slice chicken breasts horizontally to make 4 thinner cutlets, place in a large bowl and season with salt and pepper.

3. Transfer seasoned chicken to the baking sheet, arrange neatly and spoon a teaspoon of pesto over each chicken piece, place in the oven and bake for 25 minutes.

4. Remove from the oven, top with tomatoes and cheeses then place back to the oven for a few minutes until the cheese is melted.

Nutrition per Serving

Calories: 205kcal, Carbohydrates: 2.5g, Protein: 30g, Fat: 8.5g, Saturated Fat: 2.5g, Cholesterol: 90.5mg, Sodium: 171.5mg, Fiber: 0.5g

15. Couscous Salad with Basil & Tomatoes

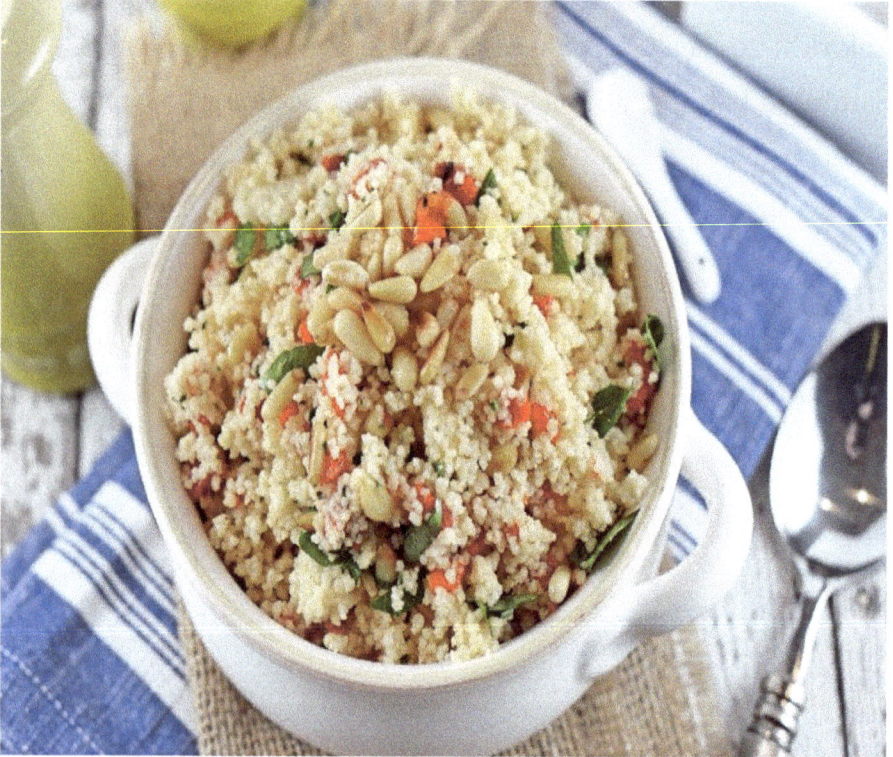

Prep Time: 15 minutes

Cook Time: 10 minutes

Servings: 3

Ingredients:

- ¼ teaspoon of salt

- ¾ cup of couscous
- 2 tablespoon of crumbled feta cheese
- ¾ tablespoon of olive oil
- 1clove of minced garlic
- 7 oz. chicken broth
- 1 cup of fresh chopped tomato
- 2 tablespoons of basil, thinly sliced
- 1 tablespoons of balsamic vinegar
- Pinch ground black pepper
- ½ tablespoon of extra-virgin olive oil

Preparation:

1. Heat the olive oil add garlic to it and cook a few minutes.

2. Pour in the chicken broth and let it cook for 5 minutes; add the couscous to the simmering dish, cover and cook 5 minutes to absorb liquid. Remove from heat

3. Stir in the chopped tomatoes, the vinegar along with the rest of the ingredients, stir to mix.

Nutrition Per Serving Calories: 142kcal | Fat: 7g | Carbs: 14g | Protein: 6g| Fiber 2g|Sodium: 263mg | Cholesterol 7mg

16. __Red Orange Salad__

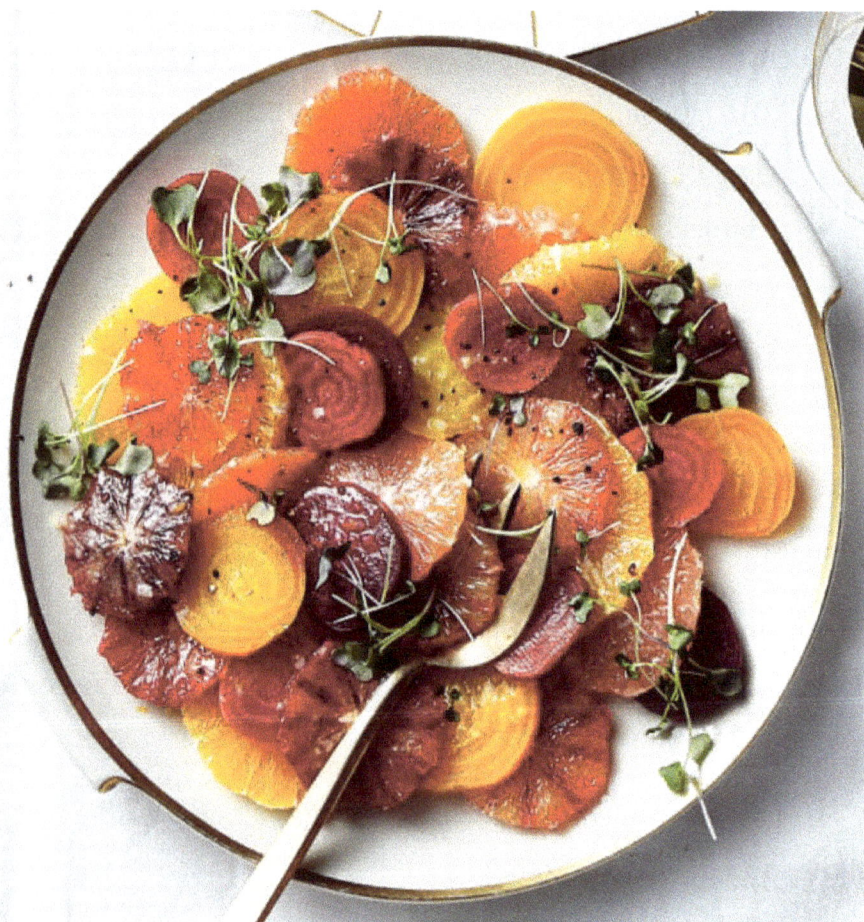

Serves: 3

Preparation time: 15 minutes

Cooking time: 20 minutes

Ingredients:

- Fresh lettuce leaves, rinsed
- 1 small cucumber sliced
- ½ red bell pepper, sliced
- 1 cup frozen seafood mix
- 1 onion, peeled and finely chopped
- 3 garlic cloves, crushed
- ¼ cup fresh orange juice
- 5 tbsp extra virgin olive oil
- Salt to taste

Preparation:

1. Heat up 3 tbsp of extra virgin olive oil over medium-high temperature.
2. Add chopped onion and crushed garlic. Stir fry for about 5 minutes.
3. Reduce the heat to minimum and add 1 cup of frozen seafood mix.
4. Cover and cook for about 15 minutes, until soft. Remove from the heat and allow it to cool for a while.
5. Meanwhile, combine the vegetables in a bowl.
6. Add the remaining 2 tbsp of olive oil, fresh orange juice and a little salt. Toss well to combine.
7. Top with seafood mix and serve immediately.

Nutrition information per serving: Calories: 206, Protein: 7g, Total Carbs: 13.1g, Dietary Fibers: 1.8g, Total Fat: 14.6g

17. Orange Arugula Salad with Smoked Turkey

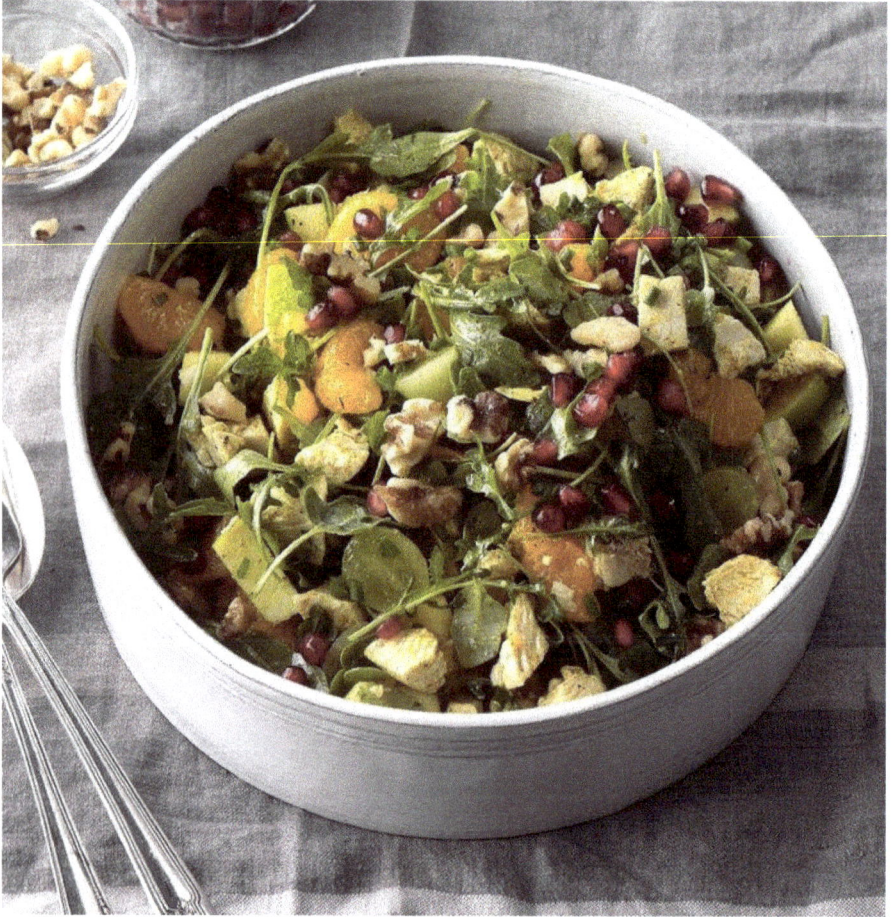

Serves: 4

Preparation time: 10-15 minutes

Cooking time: -

Ingredients:

- 3.5 oz arugula, torn
- 3.5 oz lamb's lettuce, torn
- 3.5 oz lettuce, torn
- 8 oz smoked turkey breast, chopped into bite-sized pieces
- 2 large oranges, peeled and sliced

For dressing:

- ¼ cup Greek yogurt
- 3 tbsp lemon juice
- 1 tsp apple cider vinegar
- ¼ cup olive oil

Preparation:

1. Combine arugula, lamb's lettuce, and lettuce in a large colander.
2. Wash thoroughly under cold running water and drain well. Tear into small pieces and set aside.
3. Now, combine vegetables in a large bowl. Add turkey breast and toss well. Then add sliced oranges and set aside.
4. Place Greek yogurt in a small bowl. Add lemon juice, apple cider, and olive oil.
5. Whisk together until fully combined.
6. Drizzle over salad and serve.

Nutrition information per serving: Calories: 231, Protein: 13.5g, Total Carbs: 16.4g, Dietary Fibers: 3.1g, Total Fat: 15.1g

18. <u>Crab Salad</u>

Prep Time: 10 minutes

Chill Time: 4 hours

Servings: 1

Ingredients:

- 2 tablespoons mayonnaise
- 2 tablespoons salad or ranch dressing
- ½ teaspoon of fresh lemon juice
- Pinch of Old Bay seasoning
- 1/4teaspoon of salt
- 1 tablespoon diced red bell pepper
- 1 tablespoon diced green pepper
- 1 small green onions finely chopped
- ½ rib celery finely diced
- 4 oz. jumbo lump crab meat

Preparation:

1. Combine the mayonnaise, dressing, lemon juice, Old bay seasoning and salt in a bowl.

2. Fold the green pepper and the red pepper in, along with the green onion and the celery.

3. Fold the crab meat in gently.

4. Make ahead: Chill, covered in an airtight container for 4 hours. Refrigerate leftovers, covered for up to one week.

Nutrition Per Serving Calories: 399kcal | Fat: 30g | Carbs: 10g | Protein: 23g| Fiber 1g| Sodium 1364mg| Cholesterol 142mg

19. <u>Cheesy Mashed Cauliflower</u>

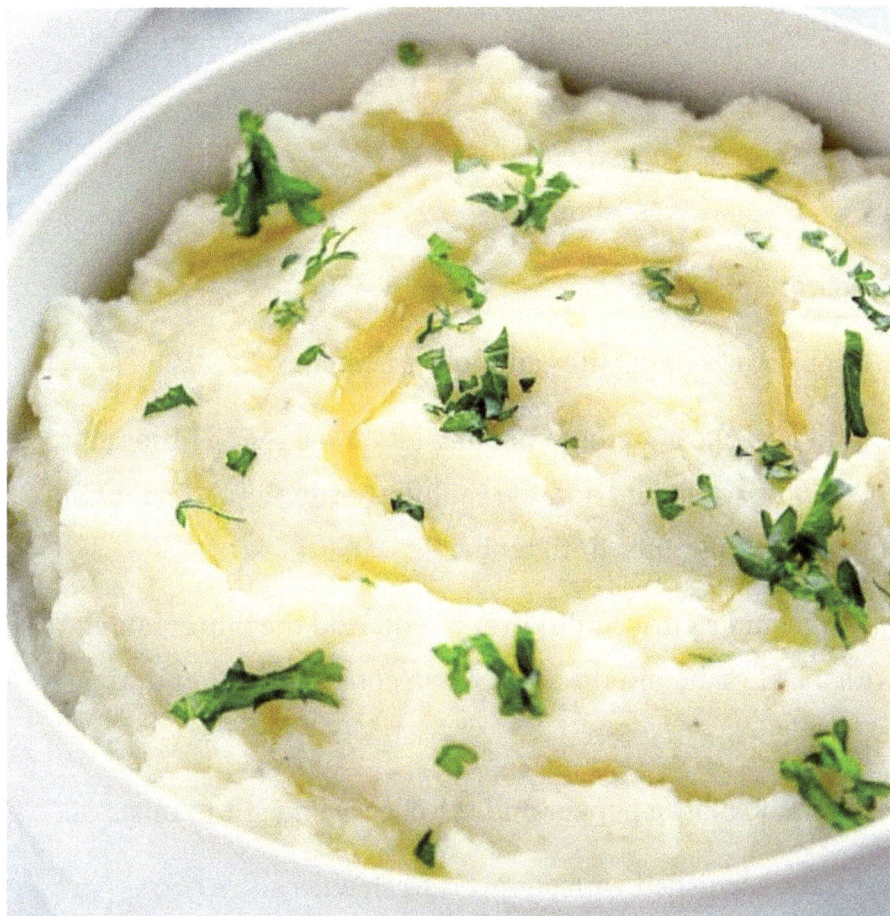

Prep Time: 5 minutes

Cook Time: 6 minutes

Servings: 4

Ingredients:

- 1 head cauliflower
- Kosher salt
- 2 tablespoons butter
- ¼ cup of whole milk
- Pepper, to taste
- 1 cup of white cheddar cheese
- Fresh chives, chopped

Preparation:

1. Begin by chopping the cauliflower head into florets.

2. Add water to a medium pot and let it boil. Add a little salt to the boiling water and add the cauliflower florets and let it boil for about 15 minutes until tender.

3. Drain and return cauliflower to pot. Add the butter, along with a little salt, and the milk. Mash content together until it is creamy.

4. Now add a little pepper and the cheese and stir to mix.

5. Enjoy, garnished with chopped fresh chives.

6.Make ahead: Stored, covered air- tightly in the refrigerator for up to 3 days. To reheat: warm over low heat.

Nutrition Per Serving Calories: 277kcal | Fat: 20g | Carbs: 10g | Protein: 15g| Fiber 3g|

20. <u>Greek Yogurt Chicken Salad</u>

The perfect light lunch!

Prep Time: 10 minutes

Cook Time: 6 minutes

Servings: 2

Ingredients

Salad:

- 1 cup of cooked shredded chicken
- ¼ cup of chopped celery
- 2 tablespoons of slivered almonds
- ¼ cup of grapes halved
- 2 tablespoons of minced red onion
- 1 tablespoon of chopped parsley

Dressing:

- 3 ounces no-fat Greek yogurt
- ½ tablespoon of lemon juice
- 1 teaspoon of honey
- ¼ teaspoon salt and cracked pepper

Preparation:

1. Combine all the salad ingredients in a large bowl.

2. Combine all the dressing ingredients to a small bowl and mix to blend.

3. Pour the dressing on top of the chicken salad and stir well to mix. Serve immediately

4.Make ahead: store refrigerated for up to 3 days.

Nutrition Per Serving Calories: 92kcal | Fat: 4g | Carbs: 11g | Protein: 5g| Fiber 1g| Sodium 316mg| Cholesterol 2mg

21. <u>**Chickpea Spinach Salad**</u>

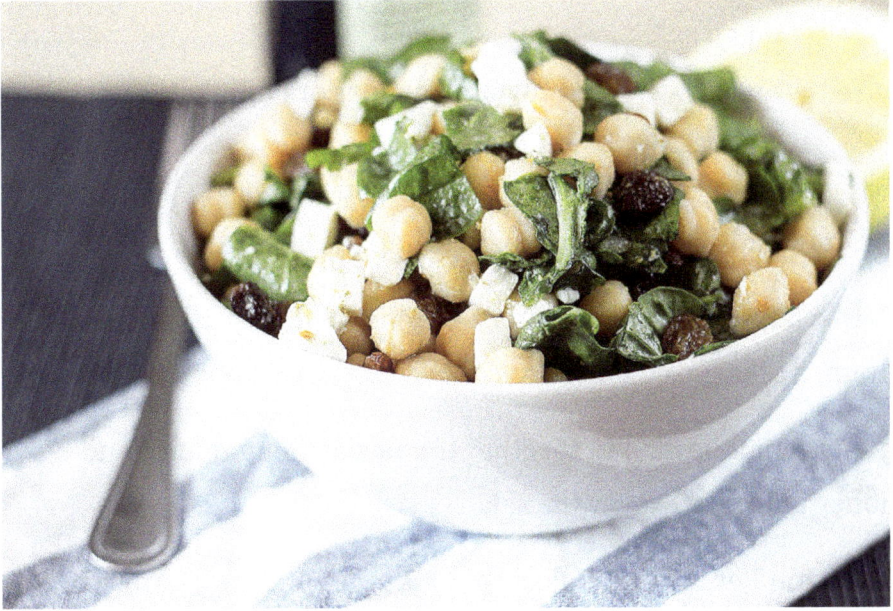

Prep Time: 7minutes

Cook Time: 0minutes

Servings: 2

Ingredients

- 1 can chickpeas
- 1 handful spinach
- 1 small handful raisins
- 3.5 oz. feta cheese
- ½ tablespoon of lemon juice

- 3 teaspoons of honey
- 4 tablespoons of Extra Virgin olive oil
- 1 teaspoon of cumin
- 1 pinch salt
- ½ teaspoon dried cayenne pepper or chili flakes

Preparation:

1. Drain and rinse the chickpeas. Chop the cheese.

2. In a large bowl, add together the chopped cheese, spinach and drained and rinsed chickpeas.

3. In a small bowl, add together the raisins, lemon juice and honey and drizzle over the salad.

Nutrition Per Serving Calories: 658kcal | Fat: 40g | Carbs: 52g | Protein: 23g| Fiber 9.7g| Sodium 507mg| Cholesterol 23mg

22. <u>Tuna Salad</u>

Prep Time: 10minutes

Cook Time: 0minutes

Servings: 4

Ingredients

- 2 cans, (10 oz.total) water packed tuna fish
- 2 tablespoons Dijon mustard
- 1/2 cup of avocado oil mayonnaise
- 1/2 cup green onions, sliced thinly
- 1 cup of celery, finely diced
- 1/2 cup cranberries, roughly chopped
- 1/2 teaspoon sea salt
- 1/4 teaspoon ground black pepper

Assembling:

- 8 cups baby spinach
- 1 lemon, cut into 4 wedges

Preparation:

1. Drain the tuna fish, place in a bowl and then add the mustard, mayonnaise, celery, green onions, cranberries, salt, and the black pepper. Mix to blend well.

2. Make ahead: Divide the spinach evenly in 4 containers. Divide the tuna salad evenly.

3. Do not let the tuna salad touch the greens. Add a lemon wedge and seal the container.

4.Place in the refrigerator for up to 4 days.

Nutrition Per Serving Calories: 396kcal | Fat: 24.8g | Carbs: 21.6g | Protein: 23.5g| Sodium 580.7mg|

23. Chicken Cheese Steak Sandwich

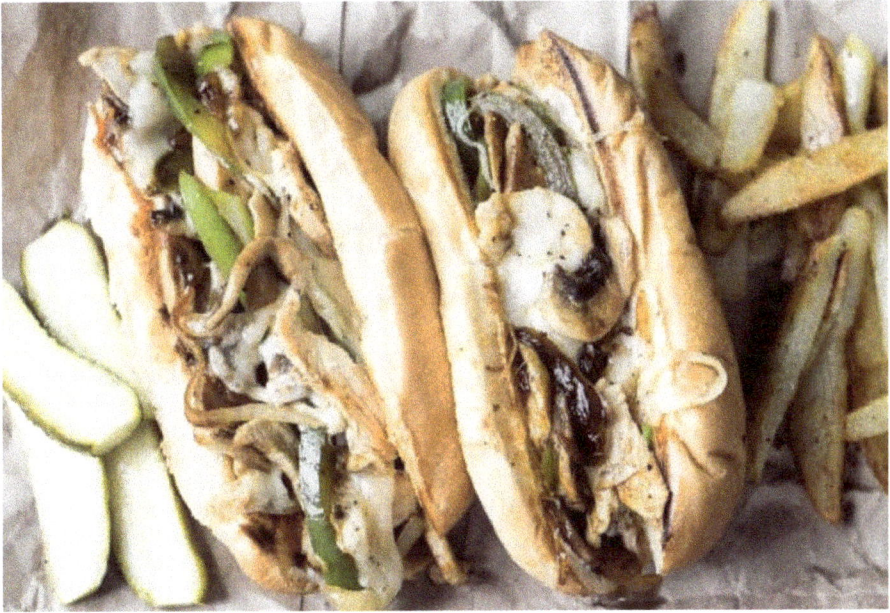

Prep Time: 10 minutes

Cook Time: 10minutes

Servings: 2

Ingredients:

- 2 teaspoons of Extra Virgin olive oil
- ¾ lb. of thinly sliced boneless & skinless chicken breast
- ½ teaspoon of ground paprika
- 1 minced garlic clove
- 6 oz. sliced thinly mushrooms

- 1 tablespoon of butter, unsalted
- ½ large onion, thinly sliced
- ½ green pepper, sliced thinly
- ½ teaspoon of freshly ground black pepper
- 4 oz. provolone cheese, sliced
- 1 teaspoon of kosher salt
- 2 sandwich rolls

Preparation:

1. Sauté chicken in hot oil until browned. Set to one side.

2. Melt the butter and then add the onions, mushrooms, and the pepper to it. Let it cook 2-3 minutes.

3. Add the garlic, along with all the seasonings, and then finally, the chicken. Cook for a few minutes.

4. Now add the cheese. Cook, covered for 2 to 3 minutes to melt cheese. Take out from heat and set to one side.

5. Make ahead: refrigerate covered, for up to 3 days until ready to eat.

5. Toast the buns, spread with mayo and fill with cheese steak mixture, enjoy!

Nutrition Per Serving Calories: 669kcal | Fat: 11g | Carbs: 41g | Protein: 71g| Fiber 3g| | Cholesterol 184mg

24. <u>Blood Orange Salad</u>

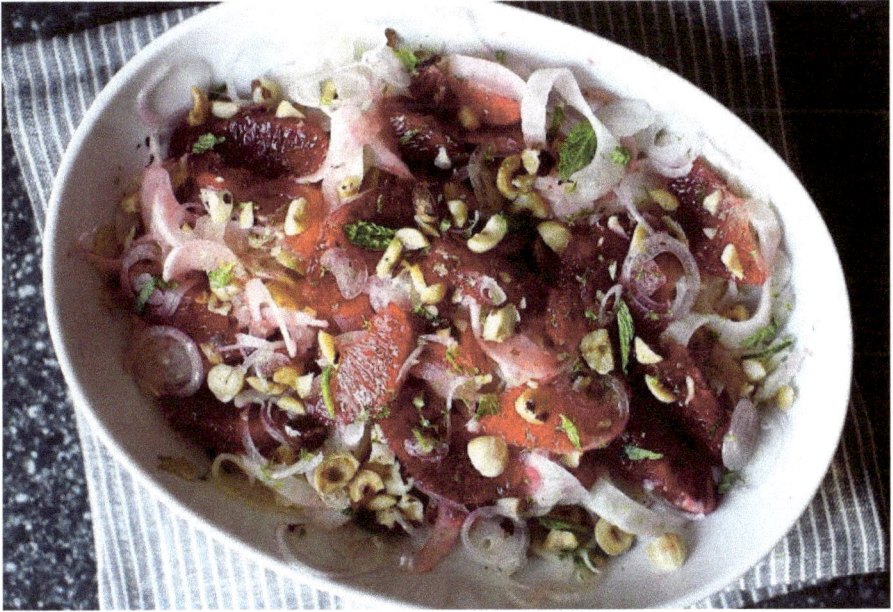

Prep Time: 10 minutes

Serves: 4

Ingredients:

- 6 blood oranges
- 1/8 teaspoon of salt
- 1 red onion, sliced thinly
- 1/4 teaspoon of black pepper
- 2 tablespoon of extra virgin olive oil
- Fresh mint, for garnish

Instructions

1. Peel the oranges then slice to 1/2 inch slices.

2. Place oranges, onions and the rest of the ingredients in a mixing bowl, toss until well combined

3. Divide into each plate and serve, enjoy!

Nutrition per Serving

Calories: 82kcal | Carbohydrates: 4g | Fat: 7g | Sodium: 73mg | Potassium: 75mg | Sugar: 2g |

25. <u>Southwestern Black Bean Cakes with Guacamole</u>

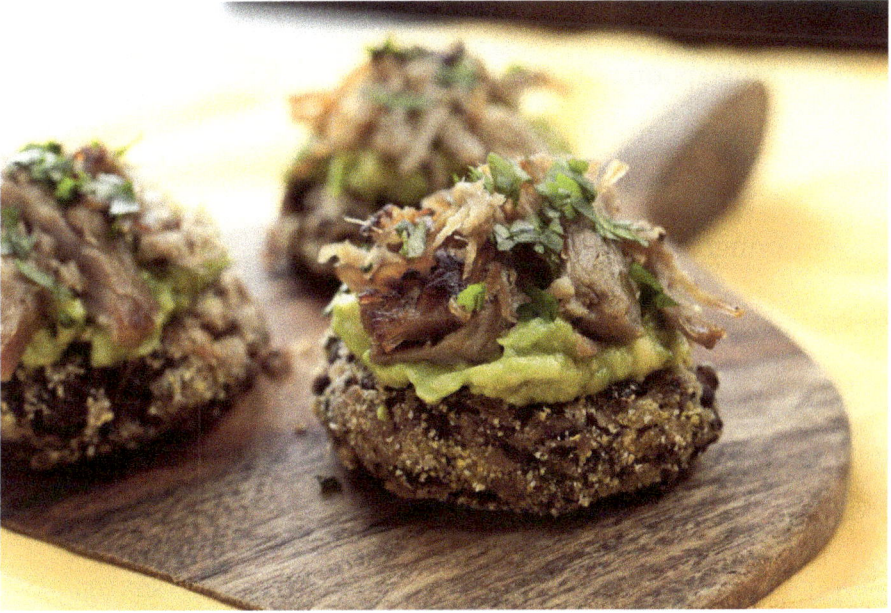

Prep Time: 25 minutes

Cook Time: 10 minutes

Serves: 4

Ingredients:

- Black Bean Cakes:
- 1 egg, beaten
- 1 teaspoon of ground cumin
- 2 cloves of garlic, chopped

- 3 tablespoons of fresh cilantro
- 2 slices whole wheat bread, torn
- 1 (15 oz) can of black beans, rinsed and drained
- 1 (7 oz) can of chipotle peppers in adobo sauce
- For the Guacamole:
- 1 tablespoon of lime juice
- 1 ripe tomato, sliced thinly
- ½ medium avocado, seeded and peeled
- Orange wedges

Instructions:

1. for the bean cake: Add bread into a blender and blend until it forms coarse crumbs, transfer to a bowl and set aside.

2. Place cilantro and garlic in the blender, blend until finely chopped. Add 1 chipotle pepper, 1 teaspoon of adobo sauce, beans and cumin to the blender and blend in short bursts until coarsely chopped.

3. Transfer mixture to the bread crumbs bowl, add eggs and mix well with your hands.

4. Shape into 4" thick patties and set aside.

5. Set grill to medium heat, lightly grease with cooking spray then grill patties for 10-12 minutes until patties are heated through. Flip sides halfway for even doneness.

6. While the patties grill, prepare the guacamole: add avocados, lime juice, salt and pepper in a bowl, mash and stir to mix well, serve patties with guacamole, topped with tomato slices and orange wedges, enjoy!

Nutrition per Serving

178 calories; 7 g total fat; 1 g saturated fat; 53 mg cholesterol; 487 mg sodium. 25 g carbohydrates;

26. <u>Shrimp Spring Rolls with Peanut Dipping Sauce</u>

Prep Time: 30 minutes

Cook Time: 10 minutes

Serves: 10 rolls

Ingredients:

For the Peanut Dipping Sauce

- ¼ cup of warm water
- ½ cup of hoisin sauce
- ¼ cup of peanut butter
- 1 tablespoon of rice vinegar,
- 1 tablespoon of chopped peanuts, plus extra for sprinkling

For the Shrimp Spring Rolls

- 20 mint leaves
- 10 jumbo shrimp
- 1 cup of bean sprouts
- 1 cup of shredded carrots
- 6 oz of thin rice noodles
- 10 round rice paper wrappers

- 1 cup of red cabbage, thinly shredded
- 10 boston lettuce leaves, stem ends removed and cut in half
- ½ cup of cilantro leaves, lightly packed

Instructions:

1. For the Peanut Dipping Sauce: Combine all ingredients except the peanuts in a mixing bowl and stir until smooth, add more water if too thick.

2. Transfer to a mixing bowl and top with peanuts, set aside.

3. for the shrimp rolls: Place 3 quarts of water in a saucepan and bring to a boil.

Add rice noodles and cook according to package instructions.

4. Do not discard cooked rice water. Transfer rice to a colander, rinse with cold water and set aside.

5. Add shrimp to the water and cook for a few minutes until pink and opaque. Remove from water and set aside to cool for a few minutes.

6. Once cool enough, remove the shell from the shrimp, cut in half lengthwise and set aside.

7. Fill a bowl with cool water, immerse one rice paper into the water for a few seconds just enough to soften. Shake off excess water then place on a flat surface.

8. Place a piece of lettuce over the bottom of the paper, top with 3 tablespoons of noodles, 1 tablespoon of cabbage, 1 tablespoon of rice and a few bean sprout.

9. Gently roll the paper halfway to a cylinder shape, add 2 shrimp halves, cilantro and mint leaves then continue rolling until sealed tight, repeat with the remaining wrappers and serve with dipping sauce. Enjoy!

Nutrition per Serving

Calories 357, Fat 2g, Saturated Fat 1g, Cholesterol 17mg, Sodium 422mg Potassium 179mg,

27. <u>Cold Tomato Couscous</u>

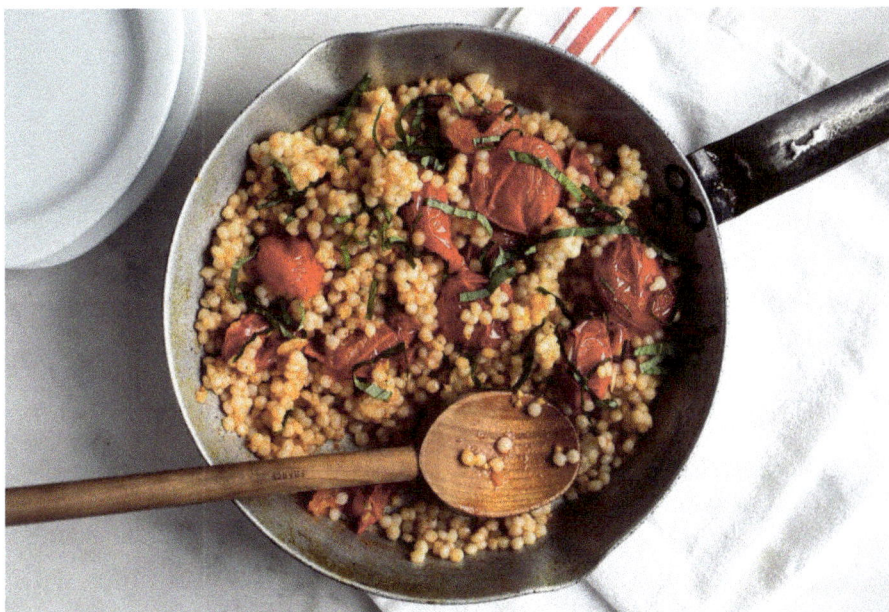

Serves: 4

Preparation time: 15 minutes

Cooking time: 7-10 minutes

Ingredients:

- 5 oz couscous
- 3 tbsp tomato sauce
- 3 tbsp lemon juice
- 1 small-sized onion, chopped
- 1 cup vegetable stock

- ½ small-sized cucumber, sliced
- ½ small-sized carrot, sliced
- ¼ tsp salt
- 3 tbsp olive oil
- ½ cup fresh parsley, chopped

Preparation:

1. First, pour the couscous into a large bowl.
2. Boil the vegetable broth and slightly add in the couscous while stirring constantly.
3. Leave it for about 10 minutes until couscous absorbs the liquid. Cover with a lid and set aside. Stir from time to time
4. to speed up the soaking process and break the lumps with a spoon.
5. Meanwhile, preheat the olive oil in a frying pan, and add the tomato sauce. Add chopped onion and stir until translucent. Set aside and let it cool for a few minutes.
6. Add the oily tomato sauce to the couscous and stir well.
7. Now add lemon juice, chopped parsley, and salt to the mixture and give it a final stir.
8. Serve with sliced cucumber, carrot, and parsley.

Nutrition information per serving: Calories: 249, Protein: 5.6g, Total Carbs: 32.8g, Dietary Fibers: 3.2g, Total Fat: 11g

28. <u>Wild Salmon Salad</u>

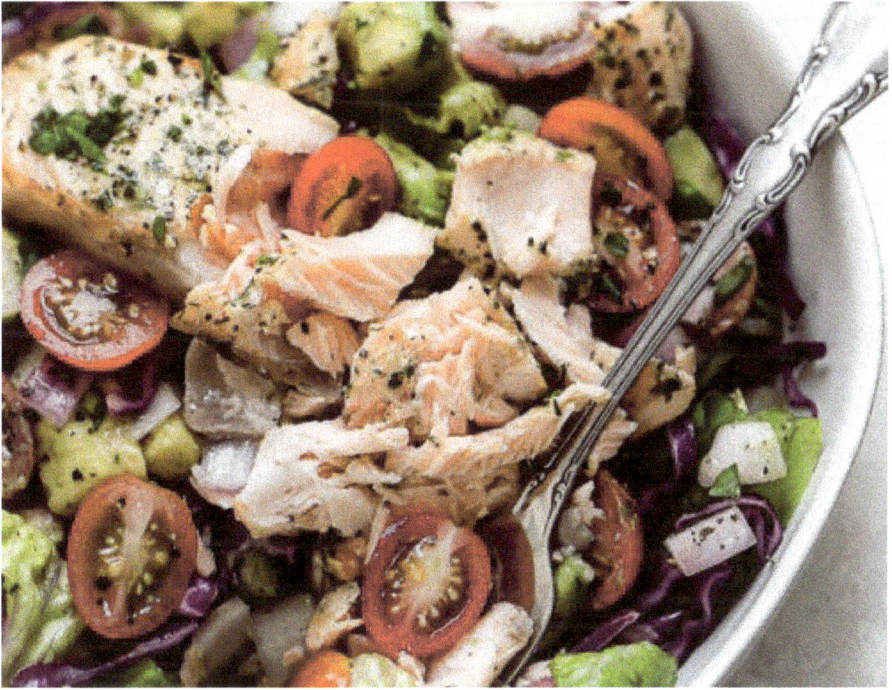

Serves: 2

Preparation time: 10 minutes

Cooking time: -

Ingredients:

- 2 medium-sized cucumbers, sliced
- A handful of iceberg lettuce, torn
- ¼ cup sweet corn
- 1 large tomato, roughly chopped

- 8 oz smoked wild salmon, sliced
- 4 tbsp freshly squeezed orange juice

Dressing:

- 1 ¼ cup liquid yogurt, 2% fat
- 1 tbsp fresh mint, finely chopped
- 2 garlic cloves, crushed
- 1 tbsp sesame seeds

Preparation:

1. Combine vegetables in a large bowl. Drizzle with orange juice and top with salmon slices. Set aside.
2. In another bowl, whisk together yogurt, mint, crushed garlic, and sesame seeds.
3. Drizzle over salad and toss to combine. Serve cold.

Nutrition information per serving: Calories: 249, Protein: 5.6g, Total Carbs: 32.8g, Dietary Fibers: 3.2g, Total Fat: 11g

29. <u>Wild Salmon Salad</u>

Serves: 2

Preparation time: 10 minutes

Cooking time: -

Ingredients:

- 2 medium-sized cucumbers, sliced
- A handful of iceberg lettuce, torn
- ¼ cup sweet corn
- 1 large tomato, roughly chopped
- 8 oz smoked wild salmon, sliced
- 4 tbsp freshly squeezed orange juice

Dressing:

- 1 ¼ cup liquid yogurt, 2% fat
- 1 tbsp fresh mint, finely chopped
- 2 garlic cloves, crushed
- 1 tbsp sesame seeds

Preparation:

1. Combine vegetables in a large bowl. Drizzle with orange juice and top with salmon slices.
2. Set aside.

3. In another bowl, whisk together yogurt, mint, crushed garlic, and sesame seeds.

Drizzle over salad and toss to combine. Serve cold.

Nutrition information per serving: Calories: 249, Protein: 5.6g, Total Carbs:

32.8g, Dietary Fibers: 3.2g, Total Fat: 11g

30. <u>Orange Arugula Salad with Smoked Turkey</u>

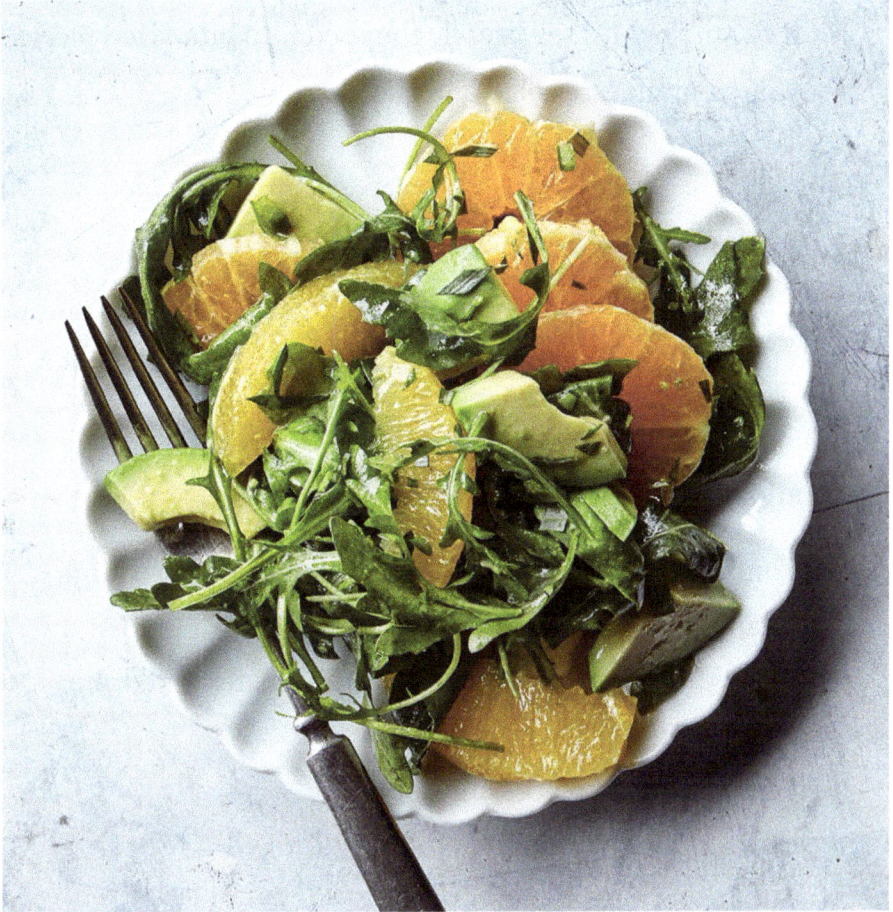

Serves: 4

Preparation time: 10-15 minutes

Cooking time: -

Ingredients:

- oz arugula, torn
- oz lamb's lettuce, torn
- 3.5 oz lettuce, torn
- 8 oz smoked turkey breast, chopped into bite-sized pieces
- 2 large oranges, peeled and sliced

For dressing:

- ¼ cup Greek yogurt
- 3 tbsp lemon juice
- 1 tsp apple cider vinegar
- ¼ cup olive oil

Preparation:

1. Combine arugula, lamb's lettuce, and lettuce in a large colander.
2. Wash thoroughly under cold running water and drain well.
3. Tear into small pieces and set aside.
4. Now, combine vegetables in a large bowl.
5. Add turkey breast and toss well.
6. Then add sliced oranges and set aside.
7. Place Greek yogurt in a small bowl. Add lemon juice, apple cider, and olive oil.
8. Whisk together until fully combined.

9. Drizzle over salad and serve.

Nutrition information per serving: Calories: 231, Protein: 13.5g, Total Carbs:

16.4g, Dietary Fibers: 3.1g, Total Fat: 15.1g

31. <u>Simple Asian Grilled Chicken</u>

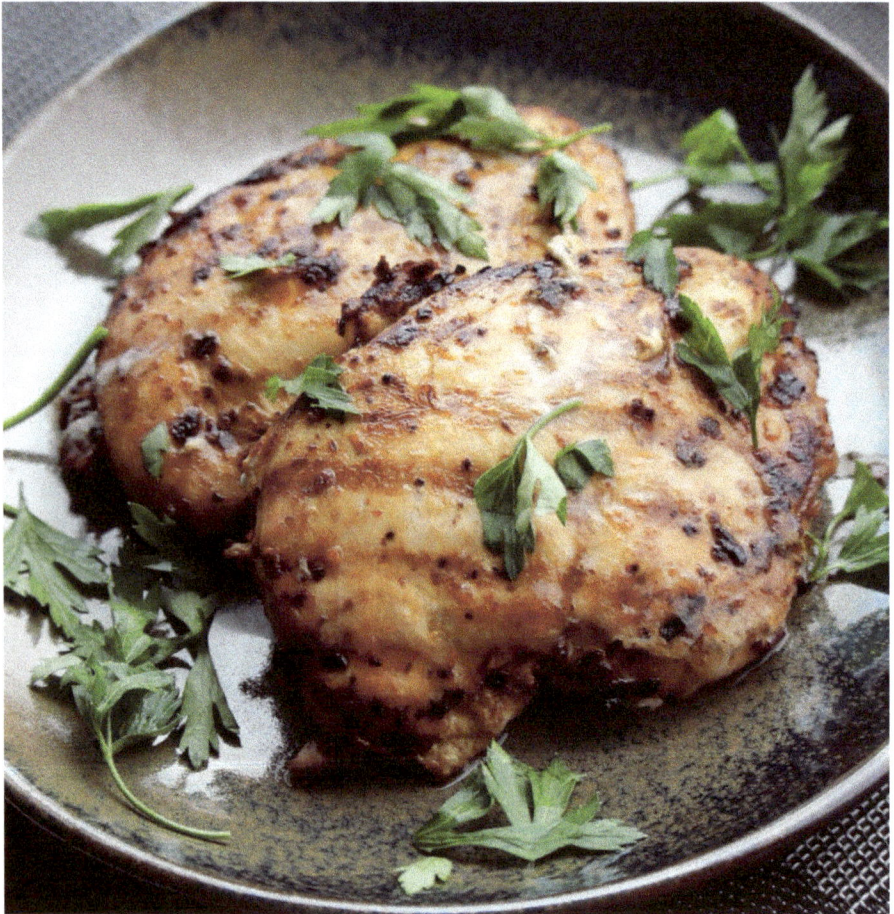

4 – Servings

Ingredients:

Mayonnaise, 2 tbsp.

Ground ginger, .5 tsp.

Boneless skinless chicken breasts, 1.5 lbs.

Rice vinegar, 2 tbsp.

Pepper, .25 tsp.

Sriracha, 1 tbsp.

Light soy sauce, 2 tbsp.

Honey, 1.5 tbsp.

Salt, .5 tsp.

Minced garlic, 2 cloves

Instructions:

1.Start by whisking together the ginger, pepper, salt, mayonnaise, rice vinegar, soy sauce, honey, sriracha, and garlic until smooth. If you want, you can pulse them together in a blender.

2.Add the chicken to a zip-top bag and add the marinade. Shake it around to coat the chicken. Let the chicken marinate for at least 30 minutes.

3.Heat up your grill to medium-high. Spray it with some nonstick spray if needed. Add the chicken to the grill. Discard the marinade. Cook until the chicken reaches 165 degrees.

4.Serve with a little garnish of cilantro if desired.

Nutrition Facts: Calories: 219 Fats: 7.1 grams Proteins: 32.4 grams Carbohydrates: 4.3 grams

32. **Chicken with Lemon Garlic Sauce**

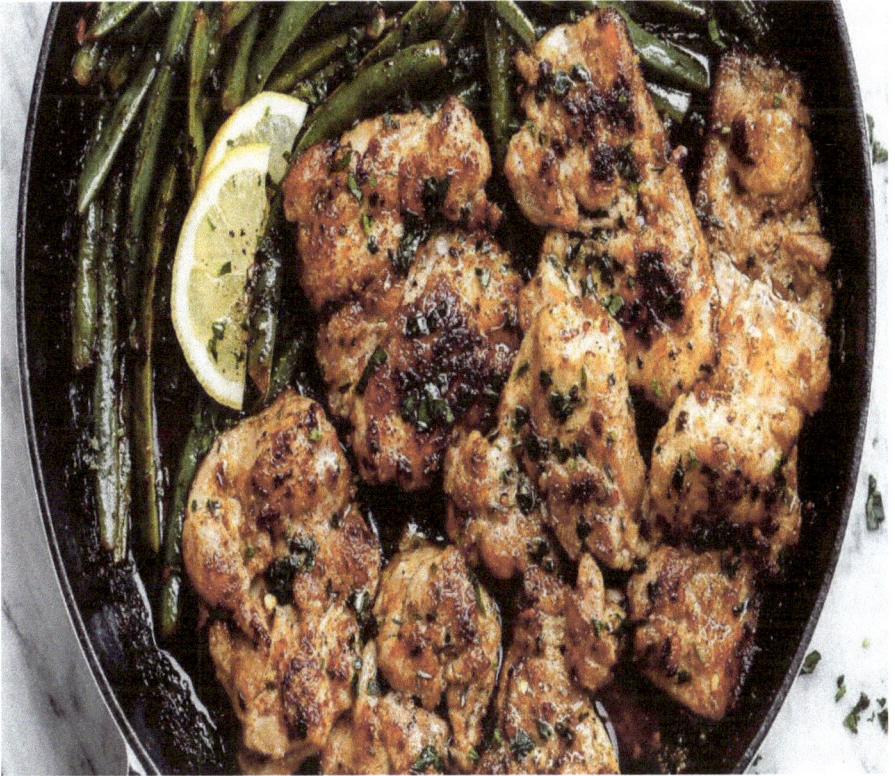

4 – Servings

Ingredients:

- Chopped parsley, 2 tbsp.
- Olive oil, 1 tbsp.
- Heavy cream, .24 c
- Chicken broth, 1 c

- Lemon juice, 2 tbsp.
- Minced garlic, 1 tbsp.
- Salted butter, 2 tbsp.
- Diced shallots, .33 c
- Red pepper flakes, .5 tsp.
- Salt
- Pepper
- Boneless skinless chicken breasts, 4

Instructions:

1.Pound the chicken to half inch thickness. Sprinkle the chicken with pepper and salt.

2.Mix together the red pepper flakes, garlic, lemon juice, and chicken broth.

3.Place your oven rack to the lower third and place it at 375.

4.Place oil in a pan and place in the chicken. Let it cook for two to three minutes on each side. The chicken doesn't have to be fully cooked at this point. Set in aside.

5.Lower the heat and add in the shallots with the chicken broth mixture. Deglaze the pan. The heat up a bit and allow the sauce to simmer within 10 – 15 mins. See to it that there's about a third of a cup of sauce left.

6.Once thickened, take it off the heat and stir in the butter until completely melted. Whisk in the heavy cream. Set it back on the heat, but make sure it doesn't boil. Add the chicken back in and coat it with the sauce. Slid it in the oven and cook for five to eight minutes, or until the chicken has cooked through.

7.Top with the parsley.

 Nutrition Facts:

Calories: 302 Fats: 16.1 grams Proteins: 33.9 grams Carbohydrates: 4.6 grams

33. __Cucumber Tomato Salad__

Prep/Total Time: 20minutes

Servings: 2

Ingredients

- 1 medium English cucumber sliced
- 2 medium tomatoes diced
- ¼ red onion sliced
- ½ tablespoon fresh parsley
- 1tablespoons olive oil
- ½ tablespoon red wine vinegar
- Salt& pepper to taste

Preparation:

1. Combine all the ingredients in a bowl. Toss thoroughly to mix.

2. Chill for at least 20 minutes before eating

3. Make ahead: whisk the wine vinegar, oil, parsley, salt and pepper in the salad bowl. Peel onion, cut into slivers and add to the vinaigrette. This enables the flavor to blend. Refrigerate, covered for a whole day. To assemble salad, simply slice the tomatoes and cucumber and add to the onion and vinaigrette mixture. Chill for 30 minutes before serving.

Nutrition Per ServingCalories: 104kcal | Fat: 8g | Carbs: 7g | Protein: 2g| Fiber 2g|Sodium: 6mg |

34. <u>Crab Stuffed Avocado</u>

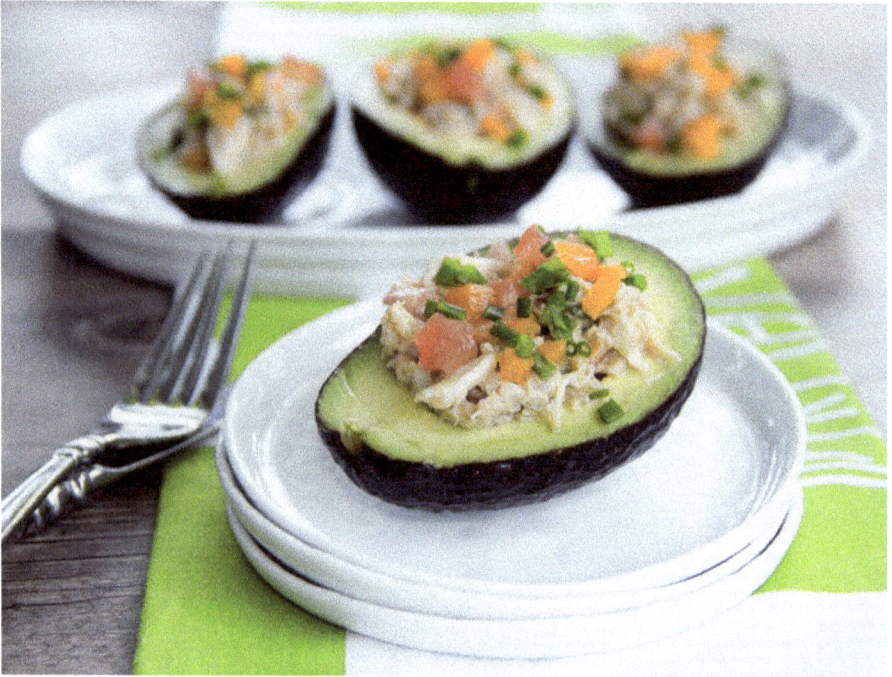

Prep/Total Time: 10minutes

Servings: 4

Ingredients

- 12 oz. lump crab meat
- 1/3 cup Greek yogurt
- 1/2 red onion, minced
- 2 tablespoons chives, chopped
- 3 tablespoons lemon juice

- Kosher salt
- 1/2 teaspoon cayenne pepper
- 1 cup cheddar, shredded
- 2 avocados, halved & pitted

Preparation:

1. Combine the crab meat, the Greek yoghurt, onion, chives, juice of lemon and the cayenne in a bowl. Sprinkle with a little salt.

2. Scoop out the avocados but leave a small border. Dice the avocado flesh and add to the crab mixture, folding in.

3. Preheat your broiler. Place the crab mixture to the avocado bowls and add cheddar on top. Place in the broiler and cook for a minute to melt cheese.

4. Serve immediately!

Nutrition Per Serving Calories: 350kcal | Fat: 21g | Carbs: 9g | Protein: 30g| Fiber 5g|Sodium: 510mg |

35. **Meat Loaf**

Prep Time: 20 minutes

Total Time: 60 minutes

Servings: 2

Diet Phase: Solid food

Ingredients

- 10- 12 oz. lean ground beef
- ½ cup milk
- ½ tablespoon of Worcestershire Sauce
- ½ teaspoon of fresh sage leaves, chopped
- ½ teaspoon of salt
- ¼ teaspoon of pepper
- ¼ teaspoon of ground mustard
- 1 garlic clove, chopped
- ¼ cup of bread crumbs
- 1 small egg
- 1 small onion, diced

Preparation:

1. Add all ingredients together.

2. Form into a loaf and place in ungreased pan.

3. Bake in the oven at 350° for 1 hour. Do not cover. Remove when an inserted thermometer reads 160°F

4.Make ahead: Wrap the pan in saran and then cover with foil.Date it and place in the freezer for up to 6 months. When ready to eat, preheat oven to 350°F.Bakefor 1 hour. Do not cover. Remove when an inserted thermometer reads 160°F. Cool and serve.

Nutrition Per Serving Calories: 431kcal | Fat: 31.6g | Carbs: 9.3g | Protein: 30.1g| Fiber 3.1g|Sodium: 168mg |

36. **Pork Fiesta**

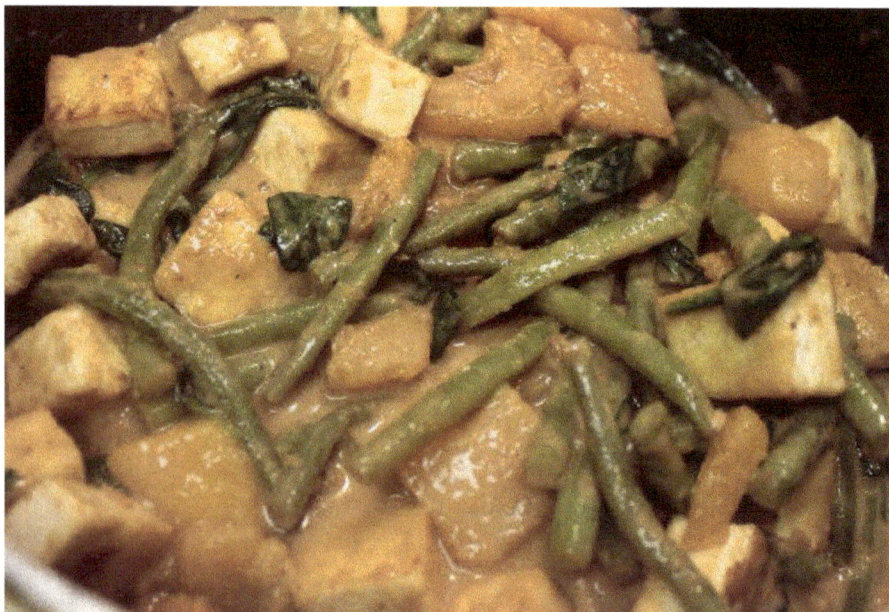

Prep time: 15 minutes

Cook time: 40 minutes

Servings: 6

Ingredients

- 1/3 cup of wine vinegar
- 3 cups of cooked brown rice
- 1 small onion, sliced (as tolerated)
- 1-2 medium green peppers, sliced
- 1 tbsp of low-sodium soy sauce
- ½ tsp of table salt

- 2 tbsp of corn starch
- ¼ cup of Splenda brown sugar blend
- ½ cup of water
- 15 oz can of unsweetened pineapple chunks
- 1 lb of lean pork tenderloin, cut thinly into strips
- Cooking spray

Instructions

1. Heat a nonstick frying pan over medium high heat, spray with non-stick cooking spray. Add in the pork tenderloin and cook until its golden brown. Remove pork and drain fat from cooking, set pork aside.

2. Drain the juice from the pineapple chunks and set aside.

3. In a small bowl, mix the water, reserved pineapple juice, cornstarch, vinegar, sugar, soy sauce and salt.

4.Add mixture into the pan and cook for about 2 minutes until sauce is thickened.

5. Add in the pork and cook further over low heat, stirring occasionally for about 30 minutes until meat is tender.

6. Add in the pineapple chunks, peppers and onion and cook for another 5 minutes. Serve over rice.

Nutrition per servings:

Calories: 248kcal; Carbohydrates: 28g; Protein: 18g; Fat: 3.5g

37. <u>**Assorted Vegetables Pork Stew**</u>

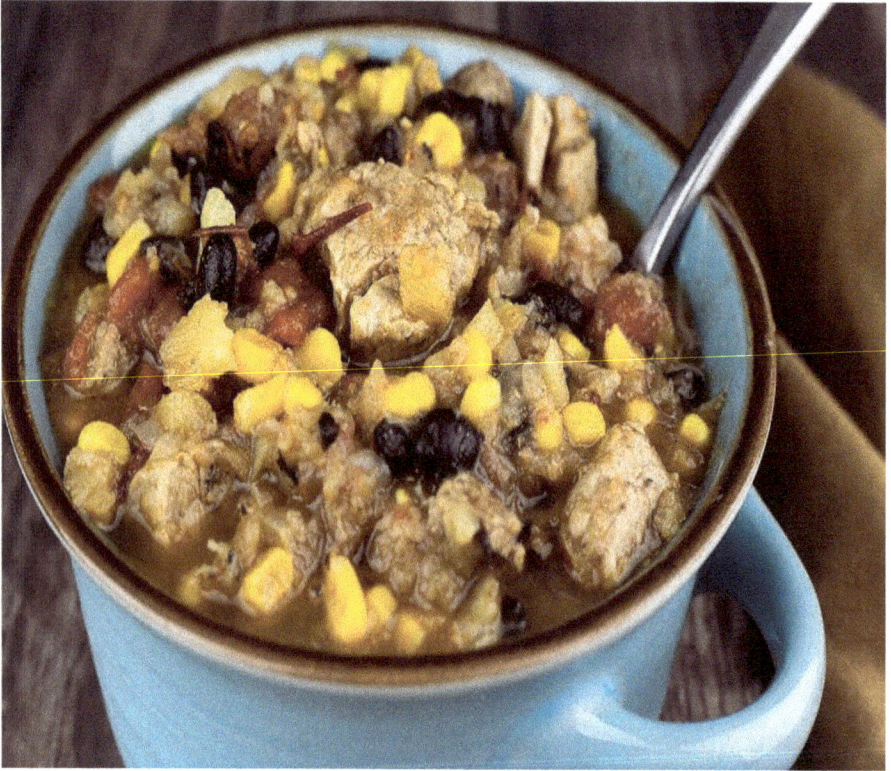

Prep time: 30 minutes

Cook time: 8 hours

Servings: 4-6

Ingredients

- 1/4 cup of part-skim ricotta cheese
- 2 cup of desired assorted vegetables
- 10 ounces diced tomatoes drained of excess liquid

- 1 can of chipotle peppers in adobo sauce
- 1 cup of water
- 2 bay leaves
- 1 tsp of ground coriander
- 1 tsp of ground cumin
- 1 tsp of pepper
- 1 tsp of salt
- 1 pound of country ribs

Instructions

1. Add water, coriander, country ribs, cumin, pepper, salt and bay leaves into your slow cooker. Cook for about 6 hours on low.

2. Remove the meat form the cooker, remove the bones from meat and shred with two forks. Discard the bay leaves.

3. Combine the diced tomatoes and 1-3 chipotle peppers (depending on how spicy you like it) in a blender and blend. Transfer to the cooker along with the assorted vegetables. Cook further for 2 hours.

4. Serve a bowl, topped with ricotta cheese and garnish with a little cilantro.

Nutrition Per Serving Calories: 88kcal | Fat: 2g | Carbs: 5g | Protein: 14g| Fiber 1g|- Sodium: 667mg | Cholesterol 45mg

38. <u>Mac And Cheese</u>

Prep Time: 10 minutes

Total Time: 15minutes

Servings: 6

Ingredients

- ¾ pound short pasta
- 2 tablespoons of butter
- ¼ cup flour
- 4 cups whole milk
- 8 oz.(about 2 cups) shredded Cheddar-Jack cheese
- ½ teaspoon black pepper
- 1 tablespoon Dijon mustard
- 5 slices (about 4 oz.)Muenster cheese

Preparation:

1. Cook the pasta as directed on the package.

2. Melt the butter in a pot. Add the flour. Cook and stir for 2 minutes and then add the milk gently. Stir and cook for about 8 minutes until the sauce is a little thick.

3. Now add the cheddar cheese, the mustard, and pepper and let it melt. Add the pasta and stir.

4. Remove to a baking dish, Top with the Muenster cheese.

5. Make ahead: cover with a plastic wrap tightly and refrigerate for up to 4 days. When ready to eat, bring to room temperature and Bake for 35 minutes at 400° F until golden.

Nutrition Per ServingCalories: 550kcal | Fat: 24g | Carbs: 56g | Protein: 26g| Fiber 2g|Sodium: 480mg | Cholesterol 70mg

39. **Pumpkin Alfredo with Roasted Root Vegetables**

Ingredients

Pasta:

- 8 oz fettuccine or linguine pasta

- 2 Tbsp unsalted butter

- 4-5 garlic cloves, minced

- 1 cup pumpkin puree

- 2 1/2 cups half and half or heavy cream

- 1/2 cup grated Parmesan cheese

Roasted root vegetables:

- 2 cups root vegetables of your choice (carrots,

potatoes, sweet potatoes, turnips, squash, beets,

etc.)

- 2 Tbsp extra-virgin olive oil

- 1 1/2 tsp kosher salt

- 1 tsp black pepper

Instructions

1.Preheat oven to 425 degrees F. Cut all the vegetables into 1 1/2-inch pieces, as evenly as possible to keep cooking consistent. I used small carrots, so they were a little smaller than usual.

2.Pile the cut veggies onto a baking sheet and toss with olive oil, salt, and pepper. Once coated, spread them in a single layer. Roast the vegetables until golden brown, turning once or twice during cooking, about 45 minutes. Some veggies cook faster (like squash) so check them often to make sure they aren't getting too dark.

3.When there is about 20 minutes left in cooking the veggies, start preparing the pasta and sauce.

4.Cook the pasta according to package directions. Reserve 1 cup of the starchy water in case you'd like to thin the sauce later.

5.Heat the butter over medium heat in a sauce pan. Add the garlic and saute until fragrant. Add the pumpkin puree and half and half or cream (you can use milk to shave off some calories, just know the sauce will be slightly thinner. I don't recommend skim milk). Simmer until slightly thickened, then add the cheese and stir.

6.Toss the pasta in the sauce and thin as needed using the reserved starchy pasta water. Top with additional Parmesan cheese and season to taste

with salt and pepper.

7.Top with roasted vegetables (and some toasted

pepitas, if you like) and enjoy!

40. Pumpkin spice oatmeal

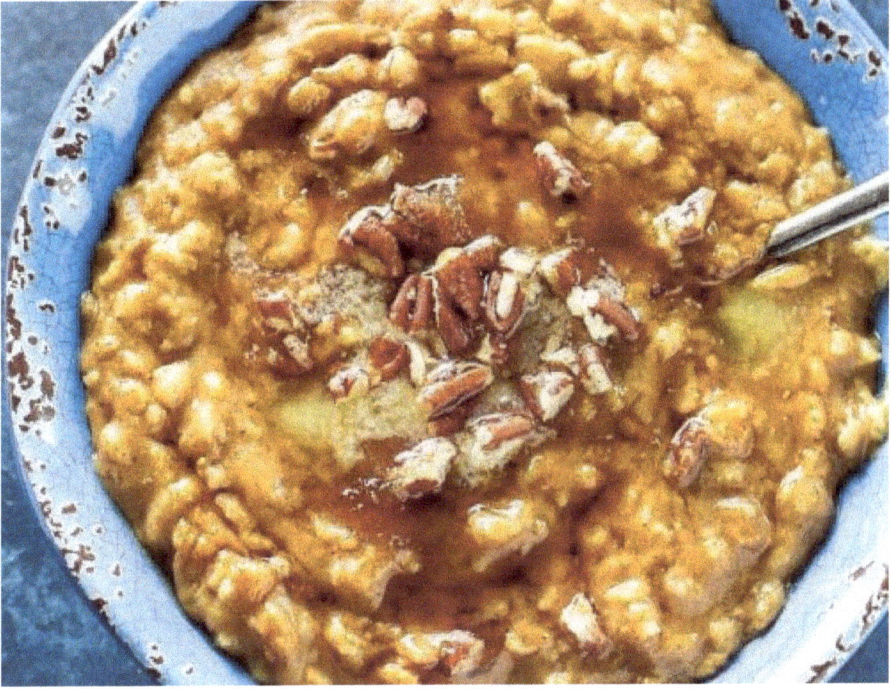

Cook Time: 10 minutes Total Time: 10 minutes

Yield: 1 serving

Ingredients

- 1/2 cup old-fashioned rolled oats

- 1 cup milk (I used cashew)

- 1/4 tsp salt

- 2 Tbsp pumpkin puree

- 1/2 tsp vanilla extract

- 1/2 tsp pumpkin pie spice

- 1/2 tsp cinnamon

- chopped pecans

- 1 Tbsp maple syrup, plus more for topping

Instructions

1.Combine oats, salt, and milk in a small saucepan over

medium heat and bring to a boil.

2.Reduce heat and simmer, stirring occasionally, for about 3-5 minutes.

3.Stir in pumpkin, vanilla, spices, and maple syrup, heating until warmed through, about 1 minute.

4.Top with pecans and a drizzle of maple syrup

Lightning Source UK Ltd.
Milton Keynes UK
UKHW020803160621
385600UK00005B/22